Pamper your liver:

how to reset your fatty liver metabolism

The proven step by steps health program to reverse your insulin resistance and cure your fatty liver

(all Natural , no Meds , no Budget, no Gym, Including 27 fatty liver reversing Recipes)

M.KOTB M.D.

Why I wrote this book?

People with extra fats inside the liver are suffering from what's defined as fatty liver. I must emphasize that this isn't always normal, but on the same time, it isn't extreme if it does not result in inflammation or damage.

It is crucial to state that regardless of not being visible as severe till it leads to harm, however, as soon as there may be a building up of simple fats, the liver becomes susceptible to damage which can also result in irritation and scarring of the liver. On the other, some have what is referred to as Nonalcoholic Steatohepatisis (NASH).

The Nonalcoholic Steatohepatisis (NASH) is just like alcohol liver ailment and research has shown that people suffering from this sort of fatty liver sickness are folks that take very little alcohol.

NASH can cause everlasting liver damage, because the liver may additionally expand and, over the years, liver cells can be changed with the aid of scar tissue. This is referred to as cirrhosis.

The unfortunate part to this is that, both forms of NAFLD are becoming extra common. Up to 20 percent of adults can also have both fatty liver or NASH.

One of the maximum commonplace causes of fatty liver disorder is obesity as well as Diabetes Mellitus. More than 6 million kids have this sort of situations, that are maximum not unusual in Asian and Hispanic kids.

Based on the maximum cutting-edge and comprehensive data at my disposal, this book has been written to serve as a vital manual for ever body living with and managing fatty liver disorder.

There is widespread information as the causes of NAFLD, the signs and symptoms, and the treatment alternatives like medicines, workout and food plan.

Because diet performs such a major function in coping with the circumstance, there are 75 specifically selected recipes that make contributions to a properly-balanced eating regimen this is low in saturated fats and excessive in fiber.

What will this book teach you?

In this book you are going to learn:

- ✓ Ways To Never Get Fatty liver
- ✓ Things to Know About Fatty liver
- ✓ Can Your Diet Really Affect Your Fatty liver?
- ✓ Is there a actual Link Between your Food and your Fatty liver?
- ✓ Does sugar cause fatty liver?
- ✓ Why Do some people GET Fatty liver?
- ✓ Does Fatty liver medicines remedy Fatty liver
- ✓ Things You Should Never Do When Caring for Your Fatty liver
- ✓ Simple Ways To Prevent Fatty liver
- ✓ Ways You May Be Making Your Fatty liver Worse
- ✓ Natural Fatty liver Remedies That Work
- ✓ Does Turmeric Reverse Fatty liver?
- ✓ Essential Oils for Fatty liver

Table of contents

11. Red Lentil Daal

12. Turmeric Late

13. Jamaican Meat Pies

14. Turmeric-Ginger Tonic With Chia Seeds

15. Thai Chiang Mai Curry Noodles

16. Vegan Sweet Potato Falafels

17. Turmeric-Garlic Shrimp With Cabbage and Mango Slaw

18. Cleansing Vegetable Turmeric Soup

19. Watermelon Orange Ginger Turmeric Juice

20. Roasted Turmeric Cauliflower

21.Tropical Turmeric, Carrot, and Ginger Smoothie

22. Turmeric & Coconut Roasted Butternut Squash Bisque

23. Spiced Pancakes

24. Golden Ginger & Turmeric Cookies

25. Turmeric Cake

26. Turmeric Chickpea Fritters

27. Raw Vegan Ginger And Turmeric Cheesecakes

What you Need to Know About Fatty Liver

In 1980, the Mayo Clinic gave the primary description for Fatty liver. It is known in medicinal drug as Non-Alcoholic Fatty Liver Disease (NAFLD).

What is Non-Alcoholic Fatty Liver Disease?

Non-Alcoholic Fatty Liver Disease, or NAFLD, is the most commonplace cause of strange liver feature assessments in international locations like USA, UK and Australia. In industrialized countries, 20 to forty percent of the general population has a form of fatty liver disorder and the possibilities of its progressing increases with age.

As the non-alcoholic fatty liver disorder progresses, approximately 10 percent of cases will broaden over the following ten years into a great deal of extra serious NASH, or nonalcoholic steatohepatitis.

NASH can result in:

1.   Cirrhosis or hardening of the liver

2.   Liver failure

3.   Liver cancers

4.   Death

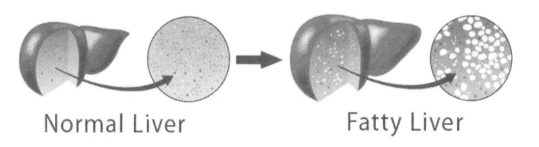

Normal Liver   Fatty Liver

Fatty liver occurs whilst excess fat builds up in the inner liver cells. This is to mention, healthful liver tissue turns into its part changed with fatty tissue. During this process, the fat begins to invade the liver, so that less and less healthy liver tissue stays. The fatty liver has a yellow greasy appearance and is frequently enlarged and swollen with fat.

This fatty infiltration slows down the metabolism of frame fats stores, which means that that the liver burns fats less efficaciously and this could bring about weight benefit and incapacity to shed pounds. Ironically, some humans can have a fatty liver without being obese.

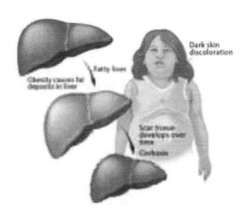

Liver feature basics: T

he liver is the most important internal organ and its capabilities are numerous. They consist of:

1. Processing everything you eat and drink

2. Pulling pollutants from your blood

3. Fighting off infection

4. Controlling blood sugar level

5. Helping to manufacture hormones and proteins.

Common Characteristics of NAFLD Patients

Though the precise reasons of NAFLD aren't known, sufferers have some pre-existing situations in common, consisting of:

- ✓ obesity
- ✓ kind 2 diabetes
- ✓ have metabolic syndrome prognosis

What's more, the severity of NAFLD increases with the degree of obesity, and stomach or stomach fat appears to boom the hazard of dangerous NASH, even in patients with a body mass index (BMI) in an ordinary range.

NAFLD and Your Diet

What you eat and the nutrition it gives contributes to the onset, progression, and treatment of NAFLD.

Dietary factors that boom your threat encompass consuming:

- ✓ Excessive-calorie eating regimen
- ✓ Diet rich in hydrogenated oil (trans fats)
- ✓ Excessive amount of protein from animal resources, ensuing in a excessive intake of saturated fat and cholesterol
- ✓ Too many liquids sweetened with high fructose corn syrup
- ✓ Ingesting protein from whey or vegetable assets, rather than from meat and cheese
- ✓ Losing three to ten percentage of your body weight
- ✓ Adding fiber, green tea, and coffee for your weight loss plan

What is the outlook for fatty liver?

If the fatty modifications inside the liver increase, infection and fibrous tissue may additionally build up and cause extra serious signs and symptoms to arise. If nothing is done to enhance liver characteristic, the patient becomes more overweight and the quality of life will steadily decrease.

How might you understand if you have a fatty liver?

At the early degree, signs of fatty liver can be indistinct and non-specific as a lot of people with this sickness seldom know they have got a liver trouble.

Most individual with a fatty liver typically get ill, and have a look at they will be turning into increasingly fatigued and overweight for no obvious reason. They may also have improved liver enzymes on a blood check for liver feature. Fatty liver is diagnosed with a blood check and liver ultrasound test.

Possible symptoms of fatty liver (NASH or NAFLD) encompass:

I.   Weight extra inside the stomach area

II.   Inability to shed pounds

III.   Elevated cholesterol and/or triglyceride tiers

IV.   Fatigue

V.   Nausea and/or indigestion

VI.   Overheating of the body

VII.   Excessive sweating

VIII.   Red itchy eyes

IX.   Discomfort over the liver place

Causes of fatty liver

Fatty Liver is commonly caused as a result of wrong eating regimen, weight excess, weight problems, alcoholism and diabetes. Malnutrition, congenital metabolic issues and excessive use of or toxicity of prescribed medications and pain killers also can cause fatty liver.

I.   Low in unprocessed plant meals which include fruits and vegetables and legumes

II.   High in delicate carbohydrates

III.   Low in anti-oxidants specially vitamin C and selenium

IV.   Low in desirable pleasant protein

V.   High in dangerous fats such as deep fried ingredients, chips, preserved meats and hydrogenated vegetable oils containing trans-fatty acids

VI.   Liver damage from prescribed medications together with some anti-inflammatory pills, immuno-suppressants, analgesics, and cholesterol reducing capsules. Watch out for tablets consisting of: Amiodarone, Perhexiline, Paracetamol, calcium channel blockers (eg. Diltiazem and nifedipine), methotrexate, chloroquine, hycanthone, artificial oestrogens, glitazone drugs utilized in diabetics, and Tamoxifen.

These drugs can contribute to fatty liver. Always verify from your physician if you are taking long time medicinal drugs, to discover in the event that they have capacity toxic outcomes on your liver. If they do, be certain that you have an ordinary liver function, take a look at, and if any damage shows up, ask your doctor to change your medicines to a greater. liver-pleasant type.

VII.   Liver damage from recreational pills such as alcohol, narcotics, and amphetamines, as large doses of those materials may be used in addicted persons.

VIII.   Exposure to environmental pollution which includes solvents, dyes, plastics, glues, pesticides, insecticides, dry cleaning fluids, harsh detergents and lots of industrial chemicals can cause liver damage.

IX.   Family history of fatty liver or cryptogenic cirrhosis increases your chances of growing a fatty liver.

X.   Overweight or diabetic will increase your risk of fatty liver. Research has proven that fatty liver is found in 57-74% of overweight individuals. Fatty liver is discovered in 95% of patients presently going through surgery for morbid obesity. In the general public of instances the fatty liver leads to being overweight in the first area after which the excess weight makes the fatty liver progress to a more extreme diploma. This is why it's so difficult for obese people with a fatty liver to lose weight, except they first enhance their liver function.

How is fatty liver reversed?

To reverse fatty liver, you need to observe these six steps:

Eat less carbohydrate

Higher intake of carbohydrate in general increases the chance of liver ailment. Poor food plan is the main cause of fatty liver disorder. This is because the liver converts any extra carbohydrate within the body into fats. The largest offenders are sugar and meals made from white flour; they need to be avoided. Also avoid Foods like bread, pasta, rice, breakfast cereals, desserts, pastry, donuts, biscuits, fries, chips, pretzels (snack foods) and any meals made of flour.

Drink NO alcohol

Eat greater vegetables, protein and the right fat

The maximum powerful liver restoration ingredients are raw veggies and fruits. Not too many people recognise the electricity of those ingredients. These raw ingredients assist to cleanse and repair the liver clear out, so that it could trap and take away greater fat and pollution from the bloodstream. Eating abundance of vegetables each cooked and fresh culmination go a long way in reversing fatty liver.

Protein is also very essential because it functions in stabilizing the blood sugar level in the body. It also helps with weight reduction from the stomach and reduces hunger and cravings. Protein need to be added to every meal. Good assets of protein include eggs, hen, seafood, meat, nuts, seeds, legumes and plain or Greek yogurt and cheeses.

You must encompass wholesome fat like Healthy fats olive oil, oily fish, coconut oil, flaxseeds, hemp seeds, chia seeds and uncooked nuts and seeds to your diet. Processed vegetable oils and margarines are risky for a person with fatty liver; they could worsen it. Deep fried foods are also terrible for those with a fatty liver.

Drink raw vegetable juices: Raw vegetable juice should be fed on at least 2 times in a every week and have to be between 250 to 300 mls (eight to ten oz.). For someone with fatty liver, your juice should contain from 90 to 95 percent greens, with the rest constituted of fruit if so desired to enhance the flavor. I strongly advocate Citrus culmination, they're the most healthy for the liver.

Follow well planned workout program

One of the methods to revert fatty liver is to map out an ordinary exercise plan that works for you. Exercise enables to speed up the metabolism and decreases insulin tiers within the body. You can be a part of a fitness center or buy yourself an exercising gadget that lets you do weight resistance sporting activities. You can also include, walking and swimming into your exercising program.

Always make the effort to do those sports with the know-how that your health is extra vital than anything else. You can always meet up with deadlines when you are healthy. If you can improve your liver function you will discover that you have loads of strength and that your intellectual capacity and moods are improved to serve you better.

Take a very good liver tonic: To aid your liver feature, a terrific liver tonic could not be a bad idea. Each two capsules that you take could contain:

5.   Milk Thistle Seed Extract (Pure Silymarin 210mg) equiv 17,500mg dried milk thistle

6.   Vitamin C (as ascorbic acid) 105mg

7.   D-alpha tocopheryl succinate (nutrition E) 200iu

8.   Thiamine hydrochloride (B1) 11mg

9.   Riboflavin (B2) 11mg

10.   Nicotinamide (B3) 11mg

11.   Pyridoxine hydrochloride (B6) 11mg

12.   Folate (as L-5-methyltetrahydrofolate (L-five-MTHF))….240mcg

13.   Vitamin B12 (as methylcobalamin)….60mcg

14.   Biotin….60mcg

15.   Calcium pantothenate (equiv pantothenic acid 22mg)(B5)….27.5mg

16.   Zinc (as zinc oxide) 7mg

17. Selenium (as selenomethionine) 50mcg

18. Livatone Plus Nutritive base 379mg Taurine, N – Acetyl Cysteine (NAC), phosphatidyl choline from GMO unfastened soya lecithin, broccoli powder, L-Glutamine , Glycine, Inositol, herbal caretenoids, (Camelia sinensis (green tea) extract, L – glutathione)

19. Veggie Cap, Hypromellose, Magnesium stearate and silicon dioxide.

20. Livatone Plus.

Other dietary supplements to aid Fatty Liver

N Acetyl L Cysteine (NAC): To guide increased manufacturing of glutathione in the liver. Glutathione protects the liver and kidneys.

MSM Plus Vitamin C: Take 1 teaspoon every day. MSM is supply sulfur, which assists phase 2 liver cleansing and also enables to reduce the formation of scar tissue.

Glicemic Balance drugs: Take 1 pill with every meal. The elements in this method help to aid better tolerance to glucose and aid insulin characteristic. This will reduce Syndrome X. This is important because insulin drives fat manufacturing within the liver.

Why you need to take liver tonic:

It allows you control your carbohydrate cravings and save you signs of low blood sugar.

The signs and symptoms of low blood sugar:

Strong cravings for sugar and foods excessive in carbohydrates

Dizziness and feeling mild-headed

Sweating and racing pulse

Fatigue

Foggy imaginative and prescient

Moodiness

Mental confusion

The condition of abnormally low blood sugar is known as hypoglycaemia. A test can be conducted to decide whether someone is suffering from hypoglycaemia. It is often a 2 hour Glucose Tolerance Test (GTT). When the blood sugar stages drop under 2.5 to 3 mmol/L, the situation of hypoglycaemia is stated to exist.

Hypoglycaemia frequently alternates with high ranges of sugar within the blood, that is not unusual in Syndrome X and/or the early levels of diabetes. Natural dietary supplements can be taken to improve the feature of insulin and stabilize blood sugar degrees; those lessen the symptoms of hypoglycaemia. The only ones are –

The herbs Gymnema Sylvestre and Bitter Melon:

Chromium picolinate

Lipoic acid

Carnitine fumarate

The minerals – selenium, magnesium, manganese and zinc. There are also dietary supplements designed that comprise all these components in one pill; it's far nice to take one or two tablets with each meal.

There are different herbs that assist with the manipulation of blood sugar and those may be used in cooking or taken as dietary supplements; they are –Cinnamon, Fenugreek, and Coriander and Turmeric

Facts about fatty liver: How common is fatty liver?

- ✓ In the Nineteen Eighties fatty liver became particular visible in alcoholics. Fatty liver is now acknowledged because the most common cause of a typical liver test in the USA, UK and Australia. Around 20%, or one in five individuals inside the trendy population, inside the USA and Australia has a fatty liver.

- ✓ Fatty liver has been described for years, especially considering that the usage of ultrasound scans; but it has formerly been regarded as an uncommon reason of severe liver disease. This view is sincerely wrong! The severe long term results of fatty liver disorder are being visible more and more in liver clinics all over the world.

- ✓ Fatty liver is a very severe epidemic due to the fact it is able to, and is more and more, affecting children. It can result in weight problems and diabetes and potentially cirrhosis and liver failure. Fatty liver will possibly reduce your lifestyles span with the aid of a few years and will significantly lessen your first-class of life if left untreated.

- ✓ Fatty liver becomes the maximum not unusual purpose of extreme liver disease and liver transplants.

- ✓ One out of five in countries like America and Australia has the disease.

- ✓ The prevalence of Type 2 diabetes has tripled within the past 50 years, and almost 20 million Americans go through with this degenerative ailment. This form of diabetes is regularly associated with liver dysfunction and specially a fatty liver.

- ✓ People with persistent obesity have a fatty liver and it isn't viable for them to lose weight effectively, until they first enhance their liver feature.

- ✓ Around 950,000 Australians and 20 million Americans have type 2 diabetes and plenty of cases remain undiagnosed.This type of diabetes is normally associated with liver disorder and fatty liver.

- ✓ **Glycosylated hemoglobin** – abbreviated to GHB or HbA1c; this check shows the common degree of sugar (glucose) that has been found in your blood over the past 3 months.

- ✓ **Homocysteine stages** – high tiers are associated with an expanded chance of coronary heart ailment, stroke and fatty deposits in arteries. Those with accelerated homocysteine stages are usually deficient in folic acid and B vitamins. Livatone Plus carries these liver elements (lipotrophic factors).

- ✓ **Serum ferritin** – assess the level of iron stored in the body. If your ferritin level is elevated you need to have further studies known as "serum iron research" and possibly take a look for the genetic disorder of iron overload referred to as Hemochromatosis. Excess iron within the liver can result in extreme liver disease. If you have got a fatty liver PLUS excess of iron in your liver, these factors will work collectively to boost up the amount of liver damage. If you turn out to be a regular blood donor this may lessen your excess iron ranges extra correctly than some other remedy.

How can you discover when you have fatty liver?
Your doctor can carry out various exams:

1. **An Abdominal Ultrasound** scan will reveal the form, size and texture of your liver. This check is a correct technique to diagnose fatty liver and isn't always painful, nor does it expose you to harmful radiation. Ultrasounds are capable of determine when you have a mild, or severe degree of fatty liver.

   A CAT (Computerized Axial Tomography) test can display very accurately the part of your liver that has been damaged with unhealthy fats. An ultrasound is also in a position to show the presence of other liver disorder inclusive of cancer, cysts and tumours. It will visualize the gall bladder and pancreas and may come across gall stones, gall bladder infection and/ or fatty pancreas if they're gift. These tests are frequently organized by your personal or family doctor.

2. **Blood checks** are very essential, though they may be typically no longer used to diagnose the presence of fatty liver, however may be able to expose characteristic common adjustments amongst fatty liver sufferers. Test which includes:

Liver Function tests – The liver enzymes are often raised, but now not always. Abnormal liver characteristic tests are typically determined during a routine blood test check up. The liver enzymes ALT and AST are generally raised above ordinary levels and are more frequently related to inflammation of the liver resulting from the fatty infiltration. Typically the ALT ranges are raised more than the AST level. The blood degrees of bilirubin and albumin are usually normal, unless fatty liver sickness is first identified in its overdue advanced stage.

Lipid research such as cholesterol and triglycerides: these are frequently elevated in patients with fatty liver and they assist in predicting your risk of cardiovascular disease.

Liver biopsy is the most conclusive manner of best diagnosing fatty liver and also figuring out the degree of it. This approach because it is invasive, won't be important except your doctor suspects a severe degree of liver damage.

Fasting blood sugar and insulin ranges: Elevated tiers indicate Syndrome X and possibly type II diabetes depending on how high they may be. If these are increased, it's more sensible to have a 2-hour Glucose Tolerance Test (GTT) to determine the severity of Syndrome X (pre-diabetes) or diabetes. These are important due to the fact there is a strong connection between fatty liver and type II diabetes.

The type of test need will depend on the severity of the patient's fatty liver and the abnormalities found within the check that was first carried out.

For example, if the liver enzymes are best barely multiplied and there aren't any signs and symptoms of liver sickness, blood test for liver function may be conducted each 6 months. If the liver function no longer deteriorates and you remain well, there's no want for liver biopsy.

The liver function should remain monitored each 6 months. An ultrasound experiment or CAT test need to be carried out every 2 years. A liver biopsy need to be severely considered if there may be any challenge that the degree of fatty liver damage is rapidly progressive or that there may be different undetected liver sickness present.

It is critical to emphasise that getting diagnosed may be very vital to the entire process of addressing fatty liver. You need to keep in mind that:

The liver is the maximum essential organ in the body when it comes to the subject of longevity

Fatty liver is frequently associated with diabetes.

Fatty liver is related to obesity and could forestall you from losing weight.

If not handled nicely, fatty liver can cause serious liver ailment.

Fatty liver may be reversed: studies have proven this.

Factors which make it more likely that fatty liver will progress to the excessive form include

i.   Lack of motivation to change the food regimen and lifestyle.

Ii.   Obesity.

Iii.   Female gender.

Iv.   Older age institution.

V.   Diabetes in particular if it's poorly managed.

Vi.   The co-existence of different liver illnesses including hepatitis C and B or haemochromatosis (iron overload).

Signs and Symptoms that shows Your Liver Isn't Functioning well

If you have lately observed any of the signs listed beneath, you could be stricken by impaired liver feature. It is specifically vital to take note of these signs and symptoms in case you identify with one or more of the risk factor mentioned:

- ✓ Bloating and gas
- ✓ Acid reflux and heartburn
- ✓ Constipation
- ✓ Skin and/or eyes that are yellowish (a symptom of jaundice)
- ✓ Inability to shed weight.
- ✓ High blood pressure
- ✓ Moodiness, anxiousness, or despair
- ✓ Dark urine
- ✓ Rosacea
- ✓ Chronic fatigue
- ✓ Excessive sweating
- ✓ Bruise effortlessly
- ✓ Loss of appetite

Fortunately, you may enhance your liver's functioning via an intensive liver cleanse. This will make you will make you feel better.

A Quick-Start 24-Hour Liver Cleanse

You can give your liver a boost by beginning with a 24-hour cleanse. In the 7 days earlier, consume kale, cabbage, lettuce, cauliflower, broccoli, Brussels sprouts, citrus culmination, asparagus, beets and celery. Avoid any processed meals, and eat unfastened-variety organic meats, refined carbohydrates and gluten sparingly. This preparation will facilitate the cleansing.

Natural Therapies to assist those with a fatty liver

As the years pass by medicine has come to a realization that diseases which includes weight problems, diabetes, continual fatigue and digestive complains are because of poor liver function. For someone with a fatty liver it may be tough to decide what kind of liver tonic will be the best and safest.

This is especially true as fatty liver is taken into consideration to be a liver disease which might also range from very mild to severe. However, I would propose that someone with a fatty liver must use liver tonics which are in powder or pill form, as their contents are higher absorbed than from a solid tablet.

The reason is not farfetched: these drugs should be compressed and held together with binders and fillers. In people with a fatty liver or fatty pancreas there can be difficulty breaking down and soaking up the pill.

We have quite a number of good liver tonics which contains a mixture of, dandelion, milk thistle, globe artichoke, taurine, lecithin, psyllium, barley leaf, carrot, beet powder and alfalfa powder.

Taurine: Is important for the healthful manufacturing of bile, and the liver uses it to conjugate pollutants and drugs to excrete them from the frame thru the bile. Taurine permits for a smooth pass out of excrete and immoderate cholesterol from the liver out of the frame via the bile, and as a result is a useful resource for weight control and the prevention of atherosclerosis. Taurine is crafted from the amino acids methionine and cysteine, and is known as the detoxifying amino acid. It is one of the maximum ample sulphur-based totally absolutely amino acids within the frame.

Psyllium: is a top notch source of soluble mucilloid fibre, and has been shown to lower cholesterol levels via 14 to 20% after eight weeks of use; psyllium is probably the fine cholesterol lowering fibre to have.

Dandelion: additionally referred to as Taraxacum officinale, has been utilized by various cultures for hundreds of years to assist people with liver and biliary lawsuits. It is capable of stimulate digestion and the drift of bile. This is because it carries sour substances which include taraxacin and inulin. Dandelion has laxative and diuretic movements and is beneficial for liver and gall bladder inflammation.

Using herbal for liver condition

Milk Thistle

According to research published between 2001 and 2005 respectively, milk thistle may additionally benefit people with cirrhosis of the liver. Analyzing five clinical trials (with a complete of 602 cirrhosis sufferers), a few studies shows that milk thistle may also assist to lessen inflammation associated with hepatitis C and protect towards harm to liver cells.

The Benefits and Side Effects of Milk Thistle

Milk thistle (Silybum marianum) is an herb said to have properties that promote liver fitness. The seeds contain silymarin, a group of compounds (such as silybin, silydianin, and silychristin) stated to have antioxidant and anti inflammatory effects and guard liver cells.

Why Do People Use Milk Thistle?

Milk thistle is not only used for liver conditions, inclusive of hepatitis and cirrhosis, it also fights the following: Depression, Diabetes, Gallbladder ailment, Hangovers, Heartburn, High cholesterol, Insulin resistance, Menstrual problems, Parkinson's sickness, Seasonal allergies.

The Benefits of Milk Thistle: Can It Really Help?

Here's a look at the science behind the capability health advantages of milk thistle:

1) Liver Disease

Some research suggests that silymarin may improve liver feature by keeping poisonous substances from binding to liver cells. Studies on the milk thistle's effectiveness in treating liver disorders have yielded mixed effects. According to a research published in the American Journal of Gastroenterology in 2005, milk thistle neither improves liver feature nor reduces the danger of mortality in people with alcoholic liver disease, hepatitis B, or hepatitis C.

Furthermore, some small research have proven that milk thistle may improve liver characteristic in patients with cirrhosis, while other clinical trials have validated that milk thistle can be of very little advantage to humans with this ailment.

2) Hepatitis C

Milk thistle is on occasion used by people with continual hepatitis C (a viral infection which can attack and damage the liver).

3) Diabetes

Several studies have proven that milk thistle can be beneficial for people with diabetes.

The most recent studies on milk thistle and diabetes include a research published Phytomedicine in 2015. For the study, forty human beings with diabetes have been treated with both silymarin or a placebo for 45 days. At the end of the study, individuals of the silymarin group showed a extra improvement in antioxidant capability and a extra discount in inflammation in comparison to the ones given the placebo.

4) Seasonal Allergies

A small look at posted in Otolaryngology and Head and Neck Surgery in 2011 indicates that silymarin may assist in treating seasonal allergic reactions. In a clinical trial involving ninety four people with seasonal allergic reactions, researchers discovered that those treated with silymarin for one month had a significantly more improvement in the severity of their signs (in comparison to the ones given a placebo for one month).

Possible Side Effects

- ✓ Milk thistle can also trigger a number of unfavourable side consequences, inclusive of nausea, diarrhea, stomach bloating, and gasoline. It may additionally purpose headaches, indigestion, joint ache, and sexual dysfunction. Allergic reactions including hives and problem respiratory are viable. People with allergies to daisies, artichokes, kiwi, commonplace thistle, or plant life within the aster family can also be allergic to take advantage of thistle.
- ✓ Milk thistle may also lower blood sugar levels, so it need to be used with extra care in patients with diabetes and also everybody taking drug treatments or supplements that have an impact on their blood sugar level.
- ✓ People with hormone-sensitive conditions along with endometriosis, uterine fibroids, or cancers of the breast, uterus, or ovaries have to keep away from milk thistle. Milk thistle may additionally theoretically reduce the effectiveness of oral contraceptives by using inhibiting an enzyme referred to as beta-glucuronidase.

✓ Milk thistle can change the way your body metabolizes pills within the liver and engage with medicines. So, pregnant and breastfeeding ladies need to avoid milk thistle.

Where to Find Milk Thistle

Dietary supplements containing milk thistle are bought in many herbal-ingredients stores, drugstores, and stores that specialize in herbal products. You can also buy milk thistle merchandise on-line.

Note that, while laboratory research suggests that milk thistle has useful properties, the effectiveness of milk thistle for the remedy of liver and different situations needs to be tested further. Before you use milk thistle, talk to your doctor or care provider to determine if it's appropriate for you.

Turmeric

Preliminary research indicates that turmeric can be beneficial in treatment of hepatitis B and hepatitis C. In 2009 study on liver cells, as an example, scientist discovered that turmeric extract helped forestall the hepatitis B virus from replicating. A -tube observe published in 2010, meanwhile, verified that turmeric extract might help suppress the replication of the hepatitis C virus.

Burdock

Burdock (an herb often used as a natural detox remedy) might also assist guard liver cells from acetaminophen-triggered harm, in line with an animal have a look at published in 2000. In checks on mice, scientists determined that antioxidants in burdock may lessen the damaging effects of poisonous materials formed from the metabolism of acetaminophen, a medicinal drug widely used to relieve ache. Other animal-primarily based research shows that burdock may additionally assist protect the liver from harm resulting from alcohol consumption.

Globe Artichoke: also known as Cynara scolymus is a sour liver tonic with liver-defensive and liver-restorative action. Clinical research has established that Globe Artichoke is good at decreasing blood cholesterol and nitrogen waste products of metabolism. Globe Artichoke is of use as a liver restorative in instances of liver harm, terrible digestion and gallstones.

Lecithin: helps the liver to metabolize fat and reduces excessive cholesterol levels. It carries phosphatidylcholine, which is beneficial for the cell membranes inside the liver.

Carrot, Beetroot, Alfalfa and Barley leaf in powdered shape can be an element of liver tonics to offer a lift of chlorophyll, antioxidants, carotenoids and fiber.

liver tonic : What you need to know

- ✓ I advocate that you take the Liver tonic powder within the preliminary stages and then keep up with the tablets subsequently. This is as it contains extra fibre to help within the early ranges of liver and bowel cleaning. Standard doses are one teaspoon of the powder two times every day in clean juices, or pills twice daily with food. Commence with 1/2 this dose for the early weeks, after which begin the full dose. While taking the powder or capsules make sure that you boom the intake of natural water to 8 to 12 glasses day by day. This water ought to be drunk regularly at some point of the day. Raw vegetable juices are also vitally important for liver fitness. This expanded fluid consumption will assist the cleansing and weight reduction system.

- ✓ Evaluate the ingredients inside the liver tonic . That is, take time to observe the substances and what are the quantities of the ingredients? You need to seek expert advice while choosing a liver tonic. Be sure it is made in a Good Manufacturing Procedures (GMP) licensed and TGA accepted laboratory and analyzed by way of an independent laboratory to validate the sorts and amounts of its contained ingredients

- ✓ When you have a liver disorder it is crucial to take a formulation that incorporates the proper or healing dosage of the energetic components. The herbs should be standardized and pure so you recognise the right amount dosage that should be taken.

The clinically effective dose of the herb St Mary's Thistle (also called Milk Thistle), is the dose that has been validated to restore liver damage in hundreds of European clinical trials. The active element of St Mary's Thistle is called silymarin and as a minimum 420mg of natural silymarin is needed daily.

Milk thistle has been used for greater than 2000 years to deal with liver sicknesses and is a secure non toxic herb. Milk Thistle does not cause any facet consequences and its young sparkling leaves were as soon as eaten as meals in Europe.

The silymarin in Milk Thistle protects the membranes of the liver cells with its effective antioxidant residences and stimulates the production of recent healthy liver cells to update damaged liver cells. It additionally enables the liver filter out to put off risky pollution. Silymarin can boom the amount of the effective liver protector anti-oxidant called glutathione, and improves protein synthesis within the liver.

Common myth about fatty liver sickness

It is an acknowledged fact that fatty liver is due to accumulation of fat and infection of the liver. This fact has brought about several delusions about the fatty liver sickness, some of which are:

- ✓ **Only alcoholics suffer fatty liver:** It is a truth that folks who drink alcohol stand a greater chance of being affected with fatty liver ailment. Alternatively, it's far very wrong to assume that! The disease appears in more than one hundred forms. The form caused by alcoholism is one among them.

- ✓ However, considering the fact that it is the most commonplace one, it has caused this delusion that if anybody is suffering from fatty liver disease, he/she should be an alcoholic. You have to take into account that there are many different factors that cause this condition.

- ✓ **Alcohol damages the liver while taken in extra amount: This is a very famous myth that has been propagated by using both, alcohol drinkers and alcohol producing groups alike! It is a handy philosophy that lets in the former to drink and the latter to marketplace their merchandise. The fact of the matter is that alcohol is dangerous for the liver even in small quantities.**

- ✓ Fatty liver ailment isn't hereditary: A circle of relative history of fatty liver sickness will increase a person risk to it.

- ✓ This is all of the extra cause to live sickness-loose because it may be exceeded all the way down to our children for no fault of theirs! Apart from being passed on genetically, positive situations like hyperlipidemia (higher stages of lipids in the frame) and diabetes mellitus result in fatty liver sickness. It also happens because of viral infections or drugs/chemicals like corticosteroids, carbon tetrachloride and tetracycline.

- ✓ A liver transplant is the most effective way to fatty liver: The liver is the most effective organ inside the human frame that has the ability to regenerate itself. In spite of that, it could be actual difficult by the fatty liver disorder and often receives debilitated. It is also one of the few organs that may be correctly transplanted. The aggregate of these facts makes people accept as true with that the ultimate solution for the sickness is to go in for a transplant. However, there are numerous other effective ways of preventing it.

- ✓ A liver transplant is a big goodbye to fatty liver: Getting a brand new liver does not automatically assure peace from fatty liver disease. One could not be more incorrect with the concept of having a liver transplant. A liver transplant, initially, wishes to be ordinary through the body.

- ✓ Rejects should lead to complications and the surgical procedure will should be re-finished. If the antique liver were damaged due to a plague, then, the virus is probably still circulating the blood circulate and re-infect the new liver. This is one of the reasons why liver experts go for this alternative when they are left with no other option.

- ✓ Only adults suffer from fatty liver: The delusion that children don't take alcohol therefore they cannot have fatty liver disease is another reasonably-priced lie. Though, it's miles very uncommon to see youngsters who're alcoholics. However, there have been instances of even babies laid low with the disease! This is as a result of starvation and long-term protein malnutrition.

- ✓ The fatty liver disease is a double edged sword. Infants nourished through total parental nutrition, a process in which nutrients are infused at once into the blood movement, have additionally been discovered to increase this condition! Not most effective is it important that the toddlers be nourished, it is essential that they be nourished in the manner nature meant them to.

- ✓ If one you longer have any symptoms, one should not worry about fatty liver disorder: Generally, those suffering from fatty liver disease are in large part asymptomatic. However, this doesn't imply that they do not have it. Even in patients which the signs are exhibited, they're vague and might be without problems may be mistaken for something else.

- ✓ The commonplace symptoms are a feeling of weak point, discomfort inside the stomach place, a preferred pain and a feeling of being sick. These might be the symptoms of situations as diverse as a pregnancy or appendicitis. Thus, being freed from symptoms does now not suggest being free of fatty liver ailment. It needs to be determined through chemical analysis.

- ✓ Medication allows in treating the ailment: There are pills that promise to burn fats. There are capsules to better nourish the body. In reality, there are capsules for the whole thing.

- ✓ That has caused the parable that tablets and medicines assist to treat fatty liver ailment. The reality, but, is that there is no real medication for this ailment! There are more than 100 types of fatty liver disorder and no remedy to efficiently deal with it. It is thought that, since the situation is rapid turning into common all over the world, it has raised a number of interest and effort in the medical community. Several medical trials are on towards the treatment of fatty liver disorder.

✓ Once fats accumulates in the liver, fatty liver disease results: When the fat in one's food regimen is metabolized, it continually lands within the liver. Fat receives transferred from other components of the body to the liver.

✓ So, veryone has fat in the liver. It does no damage. It is only its excessive accumulation that causes sickness and problems. The extreme stop of the disorder spectrum is known as NASH or NonAlcoholic Steatohepatitis. But that is prevalent simplest in approximately 2-6 percent of the populace.

✓ Fatty disorder can't be prevented: By now we all recognise there are numerous causes for fatty liver disease that one would possibly suppose it can't be prevented. Of cause that isn't true!

✓ For most instances, maintaining a healthful way of life by abstaining from alcohol and committing to ordinary workout allows to preserve one ailment-free. In case in point is obese, efforts should be made for a gradual and sustained weight reduction. Even genetic pre-disposition to the disorder may be overcome by making life-style and nutritional changes.

How does snacking contribute to a fatty liver?

High-fats, high-sugar snack is dangerous to the liver. The problem of snacking among food to starve off starvation and consume less ordinary has been highly debated within the aspect of weight loss.

While healthy snacks that do not exceed your each day calorie needs may assist tide you over till your subsequent meal, there is now evidence that eating greater regularly in the course of the day contributes to weight benefit, results in greater belly fat, and might result in fatty liver sickness too.

According to studies published in the magazine Hepatology in 2014, adults who ate more often at some stage in the day all through a six-week period got extra dangerous belly fat, in addition to a growth in intrahepatic triglycerides (IHTG), taken into consideration a marker of fatty liver ailment.

When the liver contains extra than the standard five-10% fat, it is extra prone to inflammation and scarring.

Non-alcoholic fatty liver sickness (NAFLD) might also have few signs and symptoms however can eventually compromise the function of this critical organ. A small proportion of adults with a fatty liver will cross directly to expand non-alcoholic steatohepatitis or NASH, that can bring about hardening of the liver (cirrhosis) and liver failure.

Further, too much sugar might have an effect on liver triglycerides in a unique way compared to too much of both sugar and fat, for the reason that stages of IHTG multiplied substantially more in the excessive-sugar snacking subjects (one hundred ten%) versus the excessive-fat/excessive-sugar guys (forty five%).

34 Foods That Will Boost Your Liver Function

Water

Other than oxygen, your body needs extra water than any other substance, which include food, simply to continue to exist. Because water flushes toxins and waste merchandise out of your body, you experience extra energy and alert while you're absolutely hydrated, and maximum folks frequently aren't.

Usually 8 to 10 glasses (eight oz.) will do the trick; try flavored water recipes to begin. Just do not overdo it—too much water may be dangerous, too. avoid ice while you're consuming water between meals; your body makes use of strength to warm the ice, diluting important digestive enzymes.

Crucifers

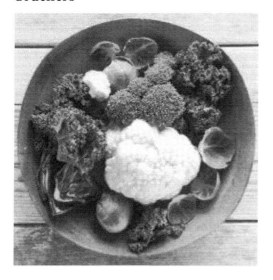

Crucifers, which include broccoli, cabbage, cauliflower, bok choy, and daikon, contain vital phytonutrients—flavonoids, carotenoids, sulforaphane, and indoles—to help your liver neutralize chemicals, pesticides, drugs, and carcinogens. They're also some of the best foods to fight spring allergies.

Dark Leafy Greens

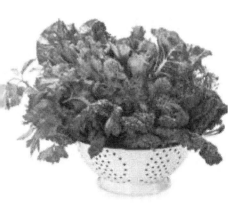

Kale, brussels sprouts, and cabbage are powerful vegetables that contain high levels of sulfur, which supports your liver in its detoxification process, triggering it to remove free radicals and other toxic chemicals.

Dandelion is another dark leafy green known as one of the most effective plants to support liver detoxification. One of its chemical components, taraxacin, is believed to stimulate the digestive organs and trigger the liver and gallbladder to release bile, which supports digestion and fat absorption.

Sea Vegetables

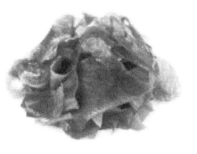

One of the oldest inhabitants of the Earth, sea vegetables detoxify your body by preventing assimilation of heavy metals as well as other environmental toxins. Studies at McGill University have revealed that a compound in brown algae (arame, kombu, and wakame) reduced the uptake of radioactive particles into bone.

Sprouted Seeds, Nuts, Beans, and Grains

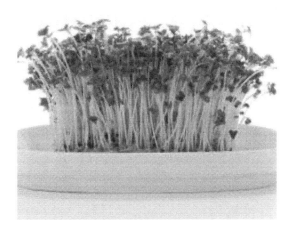

The energy contained in a seed, grain, nut, or legume is ignited through soaking and sprouting. And those sprouts are super-high in enzymes, proteins that act as catalysts for all of your body's functions. For example, broccoli sprouts are high in sulforaphane, which triggers your body's natural cancer protection.

Garlic

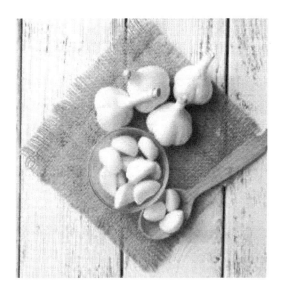

One of the oldest land-based medicinal foods on the planet, garlic contains an active sulfur-based compound called allicin, a critical supporter of liver detoxification. It helps the organ rid your body of mercury, certain food additives, and the hormone estrogen.

Onions, Shallots, and Leeks

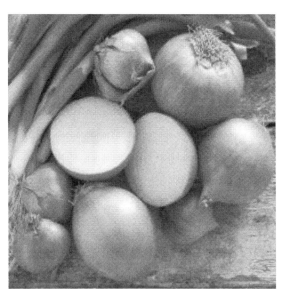

Onion, shallots, and leeks have multiple health benefits. These garlic relatives contain sulfur compounds that support your liver in its production of glutathione, a compound that neutralizes free radicals.

Egg

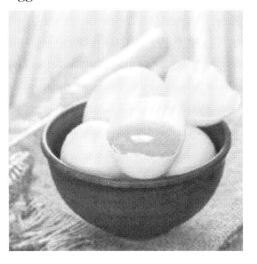

Eggs provide some of the highest-quality protein, containing all eight essential amino acids, cholesterol, and the essential nutrient choline.

Your liver needs these essential amino acids to perform detoxification processes. Choline, a coenzyme needed for metabolism, is found in egg yolk and protects your liver from toxins while detoxifying heavy metal.

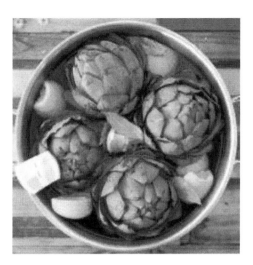

Two phytonutrients found in artichokes, cynarin and silymarin, have been shown to nourish your liver, increase bile production, and prevent gallstones.

Mushrooms

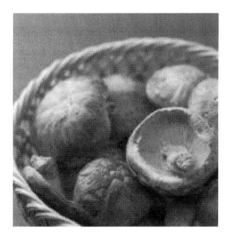

Maitake, shiitake, and reishi mushrooms are thought to provide significant healing nutrients that nourish and support your immune system.

These medicinal mushrooms contain a powerful antioxidant called L-ergothioneine, which neutralizes free radicals while increasing enzymes that boost antioxidant activity.

Berries

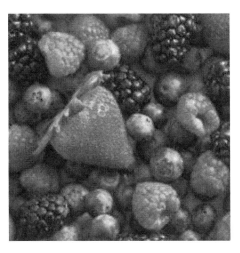

Blueberries, strawberries, raspberries, and cranberries are among nature's superfoods because they contain phytochemicals—antioxidant-rich plant compounds that help your liver protect your body from free radicals and oxidative stress, which have been linked to chronic diseases and aging.

Anthocyanin and polyphenols found in berries have been shown to inhibit the proliferation of cancer cells in the liver.

Apple

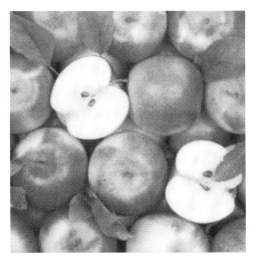

Apples, like berries, contain powerful phenolic compounds, including flavonoids, which can fight inflammatory disease. They also contain pectin, a valuable source of soluble fiber than can help eliminate toxic buildup.

Prebiotic-Rich Foods

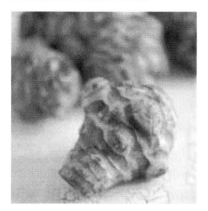

Prebiotic-Rich Foods

Prebiotics are indigestible fibers that feed your beneficial gut flora—basically, they help probiotics grow and flourish. Prebiotic-rich foods include asparagus, leeks, cruciferous vegetables, and several root vegetables—burdock, chicory, dandelion, beets, and Jerusalem artichoke.

Cultured Foods

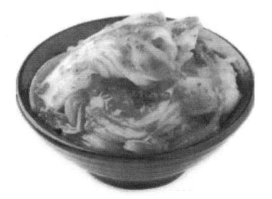

These include kimchi—a traditional Korean dish made of fermented cabbage, radish, garlic, red pepper, onion, ginger, and salt—sauerkraut, and real miso. Fermentation, an ancient form of preservation in which food is naturally transformed by microorganisms that break down all of its carbohydrates and protein, aids in digestion.

Flaxseed

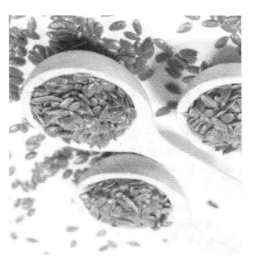

A great source of omega-3 essential fatty acids, freshly ground flaxseed helps regulate hormone levels.

Hemp Seeds

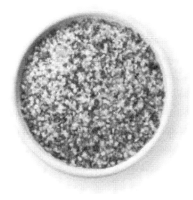

A mix of omega-6 and omega-3 fats, hemp seeds help ease inflammation while lowering dangerous blood fat levels.

Chia Seeds

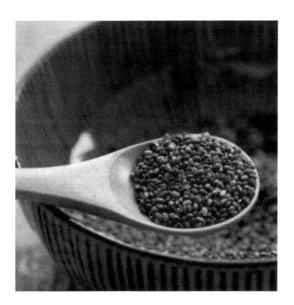

A staple in Central American Aztec and Mayan diets for thousands of years, chia seeds are all-around nutritional powerhouses. Three tablespoons contain 5 grams of protein, 200 milligrams of calcium, 10 grams of healthy fat, and 12 grams of fiber.

Coconut Oil

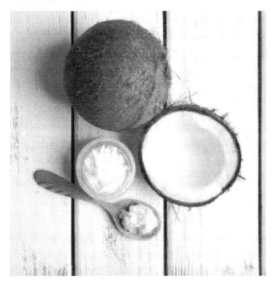

An extremely healthy saturated fat, coconut oil is easy to digest and is almost immediately broken down by enzymes in your saliva and gastric juices. This means that your body doesn't need to make fat-digesting enzymes, which puts less strain on your liver.

Avocado

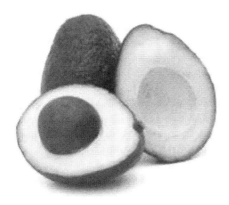

A vital source of monounsaturated fat rich in oleic acid, avocados contain glutathione, an essential nutrient for liver health.

Cold-Pressed, Unrefined Extra Virgin Olive Oil

Unadulterated olive oil is rich in phenols, the same anti-inflammatory compounds found in berries and apples. Daily consumption of olive oil supports the liver in decreasing oxidative stress in the body.

Ginger

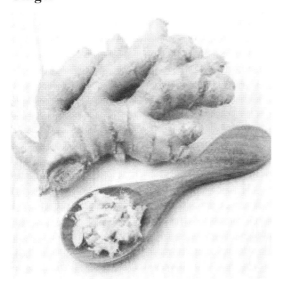

Gingerol antioxidants possess anti-inflammatory, antiviral, and antimicrobial properties. Ginger supports detoxification by nourishing your liver, promoting circulation, unclogging blocked arteries, and lowering blood cholesterol by as much as 30%.

Cumin

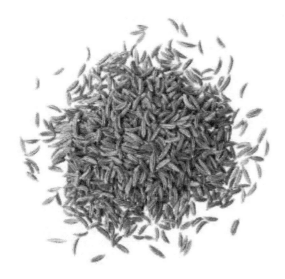

In one Indian study, cumin was shown to boost the liver's detoxification power while stimulating the secretion of enzymes from the pancreas, which helps your body absorb nutrients.

Coriander

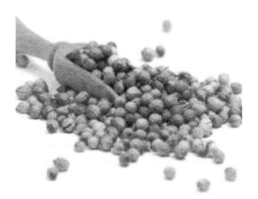

Coriander seeds have been shown to help the liver lower blood lipid levels among those with obesity and diabetes, lowering triglycerides and LDL ("bad") cholesterol, while increasing

HDL ("good") cholesterol. Corriander leaves (otherwise known as cilantro) help remove heavy metals from the body, mobilizing mercury, cadmium, lead, and aluminum that's been stored in the brain, spinal cord, and central nervous system.

Cardamom

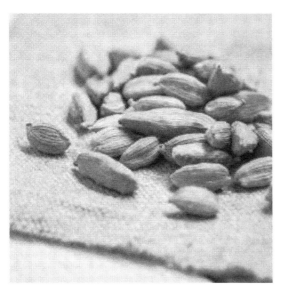

This member of the ginger family helps improve digestion by stimulating the flow of bile, which is critical in fat metabolism. Cardamom accelerates the gastric emptying rate, relaxing the stomach valves that prevent food from entering the small intestine, allowing nutrients to pass on to the small intestine without excess effort.

Cayenne

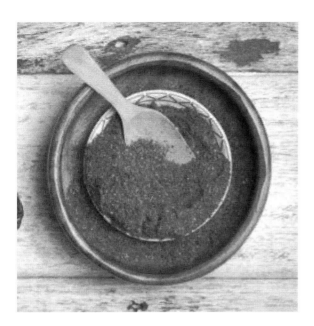

This detoxer stimulates your circulatory system, increasing the pulse of your lymphatic and digestive rhythms, heating your body. This heat helps get your gastric juices flowing, enhancing your body's ability to metabolize food and toxins.

Cinnamon

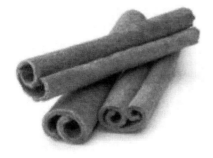

Used for centuries in flavoring and medicine, cinnamon keeps sticky platelets from forming clots in your arteries, boosts metabolism, and prevents candida, a condition characterized by yeast overgrowth.

Fennel

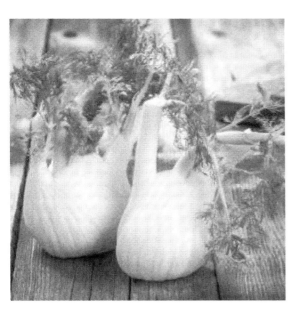

The essential oils in fennel prompt the secretion of gastric juices, helping to lower inflammation in your digestive tract, which allows your body to absorb nutrients more efficiently.

Turmeric

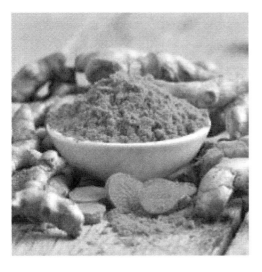

The curcumin compounds in turmeric have been shown to heal your liver, aiding in detoxification and strengthening your whole body.

27 Turmeric Recipes That Will Spice Up Your Life

Cooking turmeric recipes with sparkling turmeric or turmeric powder is less expensive, clean, on the spot manner to certainly better our physical and mental health.

The foremost characteristics of turmeric are its aroma – that unforgettable pepper-like odor – its addictive sharp, slightly bitter flavor, and, of course, its astonishing golden shade.

Turmeric Benefits

Aside from being used to make our meals look more appealing, this unassuming spice has a record of medicinal use in Asia early 4,000 years. It's additionally generally used within the ancient practice of Ayurveda, the whole frame recuperation machine that changed into founded in India centuries in the past.

While our ancestors have been smart to the true well worth of this special spice for hundreds of years, it's taken contemporary medication a totally long time to sooner or later capture up. Only now are we surely appreciating the plethora of approaches wherein turmeric can heal us effectively and naturally.

By adapting our diets simply slightly to make room for turmeric recipes, we will enhance our lives across the spectrum. To be able to harness the full advantages that turmeric can offer, eating small amounts over a long period of time simply is the way to go.

While the usage of turmeric for infection is most common, other uses include treating rheumatoid arthritis, urinary tract infections, and liver ailments.

Fascinatingly, combining cauliflower with turmeric has been shown to save people prostate cancer, in addition to stop the boom of present prostate cancer. Turmeric can also be an aid in weight control, as it enables the metabolism of fat.

Introducing turmeric into your food regimen on a day by day foundation opens you up to a whole new international fitness advantages.

27 recipes will help you ever reaping the blessings of turmeric in no time.

1. Vegan Golden Milk Ice Cream

As nicely as turmeric, this candy but good for you deal with carries cinnamon which stabilizes blood sugar, ginger, which works as an anti inflammatory and coconut milk which is a wholesome supply of fats.

Here's how to make it:

Ingredients:

- 425 ml can of full-fats coconut milk,

- four region-size slices clean ginger

- 1/four cup maple syrup, plus more to flavor

- Pinch sea salt

- 2 tsp ground turmeric

- half of tsp ground cinnamon

- 1/8th tsp black pepper

- 1 tsp pure vanilla extract

- elective: 2 Tbsp (30 ml) coconut oil

- elective: 1/four cup chopped candied ginger

Instructions:

1.   The day or night before, place your ice cream churning bowl inside the freezer to properly relax .

2.   Also, add coconut milk, fresh ginger, maple syrup, sea salt, turmeric, cinnamon, pepper, and cardamom (non-compulsory) to a big saucepan and heat over medium heat.

3.   Bring to a simmer (not a boil), whisking to very well integrate elements.

4.   Then, remove from heat and add vanilla extract. Whisk another time to mix.

5.   Taste and modify flavor as wanted, including in extra turmeric for severe turmeric flavor, cinnamon for warmth, maple syrup for sweetness, or salt to balance out the flavor.

6.   Transfer combination (which includes the whole ginger slices) to a blending bowl and permit cool to room temperature.

7.   Then cover and kick back in fridge in a single day, or far as a minimum 4-6 hours.

Eight. The following day, use a spoon to take away the ginger. At this time you can additionally upload coconut oil for extra creaminess by using whisking in thoroughly to mix.

9.   Add to ice cream maker and churn consistent with manufacturer's instructions – approximately 20-half-hour. It must appear to be gentle serve.

10.   While it's churning, chop up your candied ginger. In the previous few minutes of churning, upload in the ginger to incorporate.

11.   Once churned, switch the ice cream to a large freezer-secure field (including a parchment-coated loaf pan) and use a spoon to smooth the top.

12.   Cover securely and freeze for at least 4-6 hours or till firm.

13.   Set out for 10 minutes earlier than serving to melt, and use a warm ice cream scoop (warmed in hot water) to ease scooping.

14.   Will hold within the freezer for up to ten days or more, even though excellent inside the first 7 days.

2. Easy Red Curry

What better manner to serve turmeric for your entire own family than in a sparkling, healthy, lightly spiced curry that you could prepare and serve in underneath 60 mins?

Here's the way to make 4 servings:

- 1 huge shallot

- 2 teaspoons ground turmeric

- 6 garlic cloves

- 2 tablespoons coconut oil

- 1 2-inch piece ginger, peeled, reduce into portions

- 2 tablespoons red curry paste

- 1½ cups complete peeled tomatoes. You'll also need the juices from one 15-ounce can

- 1 13.5-ounce can unsweetened coconut milk

- Kosher salt

- 1 pound mixed greens – cauliflower, carrots, and onions, reduce into 1-inch pieces

- 1 pound white fish (halibut or cod), skin removed, cut into 2-inch portions

Instructions:

1. Pulse shallot, garlic, and ginger in a food processor.

2. Heat oil in a huge saucepan over a medium warmness.

3.   Add shallot aggregate and cook dinner for about 4 mins until golden brown.

4.   Add curry paste and turmeric; prepare dinner, stirring until the paste has darkened and starts off evolved to paste to the pan.

5.   This will take approximately 3 minutes.

6.   Add the tomatoes, and destroy them up with a wood spoon. Then add the juices.

7.   Cook, stirring frequently till tomatoes begin to break down and stick to the pot.

8.   Stir in the coconut milk and season with salt.

9.   Simmer and stir occasionally for eight–10 mins.

10.   Add the greens and pour in enough water to cover.

11.   Bring to a simmer and cook dinner for eight-10 minutes, stirring every so often, till vegetables are crisp-gentle.

12.   Season fish throughout with salt and placed into the curry (add a touch extra water if the curry is very thick).

13.   Return to a simmer and cook simply until fish is cooked via about 5 minutes.

14.   Serve with cooked rice noodles, cilantro leaves and a squeeze of lime.

3. Spiced Marinated Lamb Chops

While you may had been beneath the influence that turmeric became simplest top in curry, these brief, complete-flavoured lamb chops prove otherwise.

Recipe for 4 servings:

Ingredients :

- 1 2/2 cups complete-milk undeniable Greek yogurt

- 2 tablespoons sparkling lemon juice

- 2 garlic cloves, finely grated

- Kosher salt, freshly ground pepper

- 2 teaspoons floor cumin

- 1 teaspoon floor coriander

- ¾ teaspoon floor turmeric

- ¼ teaspoon ground allspice

- 2 kilos rib, shoulder, or loin lamb chops

- 2 tablespoons coconut oil, divided

Instructions:

1. Combine yogurt, lemon juice, and garlic in a medium bowl; season with salt and pepper.

2.   Transfer ½ cup of your yogurt combination to a small bowl and set aside for serving.

3.   Stir cumin, coriander, turmeric, and allspice into the closing yogurt mixture.

4.   Season the lamb chops with salt and pepper.

5.   With your arms, calmly coat all facets of chops with the spiced yogurt combination.

6.   Let the chops take a seat at room temperature for half of an hour. Alternatively, cowl and kick back up to 12 hours.

7.   Heat 1 Tbsp. Oil in a large skillet over medium-high.

8.   Wipe off excess marinade from lamb chops and prepare dinner 1/2 till browned. This will take about 3 minutes according to side (the yogurt within the marinade will help them tackle color speedy).

9.   Remove chops from skillet and pour off the fat.

10.   Repeat with ultimate 1 tbsp. Oil and the ultimate chops.

11.   Serve the lamb chops with the yogurt aggregate you put apart.

12. Golden Turmeric Chicken Soup

Alongside the turmeric advantages from this homely, winter soup, you'll additionally be treating your frame to a healthy dose of protein with every serving.

The different first rate factor about this sweet, spicy, right for your soup is that it's as correct reheated 3 days after making because it was on day one.

Here's the way to make 4 servings:

Ingredients :

- 1 teaspoon coconut oil

- three cloves garlic, minced

- 2 teaspoons sparkling grated ginger

- 2 jalapenos, seeded and diced

- 1 small white onion, diced

- 1 crimson pepper, thinly sliced

- One pound chicken breast, cut into bite-sized pieces

- 1 medium sweet potato, peeled and diced into small cubes

- 1 1/4 teaspoon ground turmeric

- 4 cups fowl broth (home made is high-quality)

- 1 (15 ounces) can chickpeas, rinsed and drained

- half teaspoon salt

- Freshly ground black pepper, to taste

- 1 cup light coconut milk (from the can)

- 2 tablespoons all herbal creamy peanut butter

- Fresh cilantro and green onions to garnish

Instructions:

1. Heat coconut oil in a huge pot over medium-excessive heat.

2. Once the oil is hot, add in garlic, ginger, jalapenos and chook breast.

3. Brown chook breast for 3-four mins, then stir in onion, red pepper, and candy potato cubes.

4.   Cook for numerous mins, stirring on occasion till sweet potatoes start to slightly melt and chicken is not red, approximately 5-7 minutes.

5.   Add in turmeric and stir to coat the chicken and vegetables.

6.   Add the hen broth, chickpeas, peanut butter, coconut milk, salt, and pepper.

7.   Stir to mix. Bring soup to a boil, reduce warmth to low and simmer uncovered for 20-half-hour or until candy potatoes are gentle.

8.   Taste and adjust seasonings as vital.

9.   To serve, ladle the soup into bowls and top with cilantro and green onions.

5. Tandoori Carrots with Vadouvan Spice and Yogurt

While this high-fiber, youngster-pleasant facet dish might be a little bit fussy to prepare, it's maximum definitely well worth the little bit of more effort in the kitchen.

If you're not able to get your hands on Vadouvan spice – an Indian spice combo, you could use tandoori masala spice alternatively.

Recipe for four servings:

Ingredients:

- 2 tablespoons vadouvan

- 2 garlic cloves, finely grated, divided

- 1/2 cup undeniable complete-milk Greek yogurt, divided

- 5 tablespoons olive oil, divided

- Kosher salt, freshly ground pepper

- 1 pound small carrots, tops trimmed, scrubbed

- 1/four teaspoon ground turmeric

- 2 tablespoons sparkling lemon juice

Instructions:

1.   Preheat your oven to 425°.

2.   Mix the vadouvan, half of the garlic, 1/4 cup yogurt, and 3 tablespoons oil in a huge bowl till clean; season with salt and pepper.

3.   Add carrots and toss to coat.

4.   Roast the carrots on a rimmed baking sheet in a single layer, turning every now and then, until smooth and lightly charred in spots. This need to take about 25-30 minutes.

5.   While the carrots are cooking, warmth turmeric and closing 2 tablespoons oil in a small skillet over medium-low, swirling skillet, until fragrant, about 2 minutes. Remove from heat.

6.   Whisk lemon juice, final garlic, and ultimate yogurt in a small bowl; season with salt and pepper.

7.   Place carrots on a platter, drizzle the yogurt mixture and turmeric oil and top with cilantro.

8.   Serve with lemon wedges.

6. Jeweled Rice

If you're yearning a colorful, warming, aromatic dish that's simple to put together. Better, as it's beautiful to examine and beneficial in your body, this jeweled rice recipe will fulfil.

This precise recipe yields several servings, making it a perfect choice for those massive circle of relatives gatherings.

Here's how to make 6-8 servings:

Ingredients:

- 2 cups brown basmati rice, rinsed (if you can, soak the rice for up to 8 hours)

- Pinch saffron

- 2 small yellow onions or shallots

- 2 medium carrots

- Zest of one organic orange

  Ghee or coconut oil

  ½ Tbsp. Cumin seeds

- ½ tsp. Turmeric

- 4 bay leaves

  1 cinnamon stick

  ½ cup combined dried fruit (dates, apricots, raisins)

- 1 tsp. Sea salt

- ½ cup packed mint leaves

- ½ cup packed chives

- 1 small pomegranate

- ½ cup nuts (almonds, pistachios)

- Extra-virgin olive oil, for drizzling

- 1 lemon, cut into wedges, for serving

Instructions:

1.   In a small glass of warm water (3-4 Tbsp.), add a pinch of saffron and steep whilst you put together the alternative elements.

2.   Dice onion. Grate carrots. Slice off the outer fringe of the orange rind. Try to dispose of as little white pith as viable. Slice into matchstick-sized strips. Set apart.

3.   Heat a knob of ghee or coconut oil in a pot. Add cumin seeds and prepare dinner till aromatic, 1 minute, then add turmeric, bay leaves, and the cinnamon stick, stir to coat with oil and fry for any other minute until aromatic.

4.   Next add onion, carrots, orange rind, and dried fruit. Cook until the onion softens about 5 mins.

5.   Drain rice and upload it to the pot with four cups of water, the saffron water, and salt. Cover with a lid, deliver to a boil, reduce to simmer for forty five minutes, or until the water has evaporated.

6.   Wash and chop the herbs. Remove the seeds from the pomegranate. Gently roast the nuts in a dry skillet till fragrant and golden.

7.	When the rice is cooked, cast off from the warmth. Scoop rice out onto a baking sheet to cool barely and to save you the grains from sticking together.

8.	Wait a couple of minutes before sprinkling with herbs, nuts, and pomegranate seeds. Fold to contain.

9.	Season to flavor and revel in.

7. Yellow Chicken Adobo

This national dish of the Philippines will really provide you along with your recommended day by day quantity of turmeric. And even though you'll want a few 'unique device' (inside the shape of a layer of cheesecloth) it's worth it.

Here's a way to make it:

Ingredients:

- 10 dried bay leaves

- 2 tablespoons black peppercorns

- 2 tablespoons floor turmeric

- 1/four cup unsweetened shredded coconut

- half head of cauliflower, damaged into small florets

- 1/four kabocha squash, cut into 1-inch pieces (about 2 cups)

- 3 tablespoons vegetable oil, divided

- Kosher salt, freshly floor pepper

- 1 small white onion, chopped

- 2 medium shallots, chopped

- 6 huge garlic cloves, chopped

- 1 (3-inch) piece ginger, peeled, finely grated

- 1 teaspoon crushed pink pepper flakes

- 2 (13.Five-ounce) cans unsweetened coconut milk

- 1 cup sugarcane vinegar or distilled white vinegar, divided

- four chook legs, drumsticks, and thighs, separated

- 3 tablespoons honey

- Unsalted, roasted pumpkin seeds, thinly sliced Fresno chiles, and sliced scallion (for serving)

- A layer of cheesecloth

Instructions:

1. Place bay leaves and peppercorns inside the middle of a cheesecloth and tie it closed with kitchen wire. Set aside.

2. Toast turmeric in a dry small skillet over a medium-low warmness. Stir regularly, just ill aromatic. Don't allow it brown. This will take approximately three minutes. Transfer to a plate.

3. Cook coconut in the same skillet over medium-excessive warmth, stirring occasionally, until brown.This will take about three minutes. Grind in a spice mill or with a mortar and pestle or finely chop.

4. Transfer to any other plate.

5. Heat your oven to 375°F. Toss cauliflower and squash on a huge rimmed baking sheet with 1 Tbsp of oil to coat; season with salt and pepper.

6. Roast the greens for approximately 30-forty minutes, tossing on occasion, till browned and gentle.

7. Heat last 2 tbsp. Oil in a massive Dutch oven or other heavy pot over medium-high. Add onion, shallots, garlic, and ginger and prepare dinner, stirring frequently, until golden brown and really aromatic, 8–10 minutes.

8.   Add purple pepper flakes and cook, stirring frequently, simply until aromatic, about 1 minute.

9.   Stir in toasted turmeric, coconut milk, and three/four cup vinegar. Bring to a boil and prepare dinner until liquid is reduced by means of about one-1/3, 20–30 minutes.

10.   Prepare a grill for medium-excessive heat (or heat a grill pan over medium-high). Season hen with salt and pepper and grill, turning occasionally, simply till pores and skin is charred (chicken will not be cooked via at this factor), 8–10 mins.

11.   Add fowl and reserved sachet to turmeric sauce. Cook, partially covered, until chook is gentle, 60–eighty mins.

12.   Stir honey and remaining 1/4 cup vinegar in a small bowl till honey is dissolved; upload to braise, then add roasted cauliflower and squash. Taste and season with extra salt or honey as needed.

13.   To serve, divide the adobo amongst bowls and top with burnt coconut, pumpkin seeds, chiles, and scallion.

8. Grilled Clams With Aleppo Pepper, Turmeric, And Lime Butter

In case you have been questioning if you can deliver turmeric to the BBQ… the answer is sure! It works beautifully blended with pepper, lime, and butter and served with grilled clams.

To make 4 servings:

Ingredients:

- ½ cup (1 stick) unsalted butter, room temperature

- 2 teaspoons Aleppo pepper or 1 crushed red pepper flakes

- 1 teaspoon finely grated peeled turmeric or ½ ground dried turmeric

- 1 teaspoon finely grated lime zest

- Kosher salt

- Grilled clams

Instructions:

1.   Place butter, Aleppo pepper, and turmeric in a small bowl.

2.   Add lime zest and blend until well mixed; season with salt.

Three. Add butter to bowl with grilled clams and toss to coat.

Four.   Transfer to a serving platter and pinnacle with cilantro to serve.

9. Miso-Turmeric Dressing

If you're looking for a speedy manner to get your turmeric dose, do this dressing on salmon or noodles. You really can't pass wrong with it!

Here's the recipe for 1 cup:

Ingredients:

- 1/3 cup rice vinegar

- 1/four cup mirin

- 1/4 cup vegetable oil

- 2 tablespoons finely grated carrot

- 2 tablespoons white miso

- 1 tablespoon finely grated peeled ginger

- 2 teaspoons finely grated peeled turmeric

- 1 teaspoon toasted sesame oil

Instructions:

1.   Whisk vinegar, mirin, vegetable oil, carrot, miso, ginger, turmeric, and sesame oil in a small bowl.

2.   Serve over seared salmon or cooked soba noodles.

10. Honey-Turmeric Beef with Beet and Carrot Salad

Here's a way to make 4 servings:

Ingredients:

- 1¼ kilos boneless red meat shoulder, fats trimmed and reduce into four pieces

- Kosher salt and freshly floor black pepper

- 2 garlic cloves, finely grated

- 1½ teaspoons finely grated peeled turmeric or ½ floor turmeric

- ½ cup plain yogurt

- ¼ cup honey

- 2 tablespoons (or greater) clean lemon juice, divided

- 2 tablespoons vegetable oil

- 3 small beets, scrubbed, thinly sliced

- three small carrots, preferably with tops, tops reserved, carrots scrubbed, cut on a diagonal

- 2 tablespoons finely chopped fresh chives

- 2 tablespoons olive oil

- Himalayan salt

Instructions:

1.   Pound red meat between 2 sheets of plastic wrap to ¼" thick; season with kosher salt and pepper.

2.   Whisk garlic, turmeric, yogurt, honey, and 1 tbsp. Lemon juice in a small bowl; season with kosher salt and pepper.

3.   Place cutlets in a large resealable bag. Add yogurt combination, seal bag, and toss to coat. Let sit down at the least 10 minutes.

4.   Remove cutlets from marinade, letting excess drip off.

5.   Heat 1 tbsp. Vegetable oil in a large skillet over medium-high; cook 2 cutlets until browned and cooked via, about 2 minutes in step with facet.

6.   Transfer red meat to a platter. Wipe out skillet; repeat with last cutlets and 1 Tbsp. Vegetable oil.

7.   Toss beets, carrots, carrot tops (if the use of), chives, olive oil, and remaining 1 tbsp. Lemon juice in a small bowl.

8.   Season with kosher salt, pepper, and extra lemon juice, if preferred.

9.   Sprinkled with sea salt and serve heat.

11. Red Lentil Daal

For a brief, healthful yet comforting dinner, daal is an excellent desire. Using lots of heat and peppery turmeric is a notable opportunity to piling at the salt.

Serves three

Ingredients:

- 2 cups pink lentils

- ½ cup coconut milk

- 2 cups hot water

- 1-inch ginger piece, peeled and grated

- 1 onion, finely diced

- 2 garlic cloves, overwhelmed

- 1 tsp coconut oil

- 1 tsp turmeric powder

- ½ tsp garam masala

- Coconut milk, blended seeds. And clean parsley leaves, to garnish

- ½ tsp Himalayan salt

- Freshly floor black pepper

Instructions:

1.	Rinse the pink lentils with bloodless water and drain.

2.	In a medium saucepan heat the coconut oil, upload the onion, garlic, ginger, and turmeric, and cook for 2 mins, stirring regularly.

3.	Add the lentils and water, bring to boil and allow simmer for 15 minutes.

4.	Add garam masala and coconut milk and blend to combine.

5.	Let simmer for any other five minutes, till all of the liquid is absorbed.

6.	Serve the daal warm, garnished with a few drops of coconut milk.

12. Turmeric Late

If you're a coffee lover, this healthy latte – sure, you read that right- is stuffed with turmeric. It may be the ideal substitute in your caffeinated indulgence.

Here's how to make it:

Ingredients:

- ½ cup coconut milk

- 1 tablespoon date sugar or 2 teaspoons raw sugar

- four teaspoons freshly grated turmeric or 1 teaspoon floor turmeric

- 1 teaspoon freshly grated ginger or ¼ teaspoon ground ginger

- ⅛ teaspoon Chinese 5-spice powder or floor nutmeg

- Pinch of kosher salt

Instructions:

1.   Whisk coconut milk, sugar, turmeric, ginger, five-spice, salt, and ¾ cup water in a small saucepan and produce to a boil.

2.   Remove from heat and let combination steep 5 minutes. Strain through a great-mesh sieve into a mug and serve.

13. Jamaican Meat Pies

These unique Jamaican meat pies are specific in their taste and shade because of the addition of turmeric.

To make 10-12 servings:

Ingredients:

For the crust

- four cups unbleached all-purpose flour (plus greater for dusting)

- 2 tablespoon coconut sugar

- ½ tablespoon salt

- ½ – 2-teaspoon turmeric

- 10 ounces. Butter

- 1 tablespoon apple cider vinegar

- 1 cup iced water

For the filling

- 1 teaspoon curry

- ½ medium onion chopped

- 1 teaspoon minced garlic

- 1 teaspoon paprika

- ½ teaspoon all spice powder

- 1 teaspoon dried thyme

- 1 teaspoon white pepper

- 3 green onion, chopped

- 2 tablespoon chopped parsley

- 1 ½ teaspoon salt or greater

- ½ teaspoon chili pepper

- 1 pound floor red meat

- ¼ cup bread crumbs

- ½ scotch bonnet pepper chopped (non-compulsory)

Instructions:

1.   In a food processor or by using hand, blend together, flour, salt, sugar, turmeric blend well

2.   Add the butter, followed through vinegar and water in small quantities, pulse until combined and dough holds together in a ball.

3.   Place the dough on a properly-floured surface. Divide it into 2 and roll it out.

4.   Place within the refrigerator for as a minimum 30 minutes till equipped to use

5.   While you wait, prepare the filling through add 2 tablespoons of oil to a saucepan, followed by using onions, garlic, paprika, thyme curry, chili powder, white pepper, and all spice. Let it simmer for about 2 minutes,

6.   Then, upload floor meat, bread crumbs and maintain cooking for approximately 10 or extra mins.Stirring often to prevent burning, upload about ½ cup of water.

7.   Finally upload green onions and parsley, alter for salt and pepper seasoning.

8.   Remove from stovetop and permit it cool.

9.   Using a massive mouth, glass or bowl about four – 5 " cut out circles by using gently pressing at the dough and releasing it, shaping the meat pie dough. Continue slicing out dough till all dough has been reduce.

10.   Refrigerate until equipped to apply.

11.   Scoop a heaping tablespoon of filling into each circle, and brush with egg white or white round half of of the circle. Fold over twist with fingers lightly to seal the rims of the meat pie.

12.   Another way of sealing is by means of urgent the tines of a fork alongside the edges of the dough.

13.   Carefully region every pie on a baking sheet and bake for approximately 30 minutes.

14.   Serve warm. Leftovers may be frozen.

14. Turmeric-Ginger Tonic With Chia Seeds

This sparkling and turmeric tonic is not for the faint hearted! Be prepared for the heat from the turmeric and peppercorns.

Here's the way to make for four servings:

Ingredients:

- 1 4-inch piece peeled ginger, coarsely chopped

- 1 four-inch piece peeled turmeric, coarsely chopped

- ⅓ cup honey

- ¼ cup sparkling lime juice

- 2 teaspoons black peppercorns

- 1 tablespoon chia seeds

Instructions:

1. Blend ginger, turmeric, honey, lime juice, black peppercorns, and 3 cups water in a food processor

2. Until smooth.

3. Strain thru a excellent-mesh sieve right into a big bowl. Stir in chia seeds and let take a seat till seeds start to swell. This will take about eight–10 mins.

4- Divide the tonic among ice-crammed glasses.

5- Drink at once.

15. Thai Chiang Mai Curry Noodles

As tastes nicely because of the turmeric, this recipe is full of lots of other accurate-for-you substances. This dish from Northern Thailand is generally served up in a giant bowl.

Here's the recipe for six servings:

Ingredients:

- 2 tablespoons vegetable oil

- 1 tablespoon finely chopped garlic

- 2 tablespoons pink curry paste or 2 tablespoons Panang curry paste

- three⁄4 lb boneless chicken, cut into huge bite-sized chunks along with tri-tip steak or 3⁄4

- lb flank steak, thinly sliced crosswise into 2-inch strips

- 2 cups unsweetened coconut milk

- 1 three⁄four cups fowl broth

- 2 teaspoons ground turmeric or 2 teaspoons curry powder

- 2 tablespoons soy sauce

- 1 teaspoon sugar

- 1 teaspoon salt

- 1⁄3 cup coarsely chopped shallots

- 2 tablespoons freshly squeezed lime juice

- 1⁄three cup coarsely chopped fresh cilantro

- 1⁄three cup thinly sliced inexperienced onion

- 1 lb fresh Chinese noodles

Instructions:

1. Heat the vegetable oil in a medium saucepan over medium warmth, after which add the garlic. Toss properly and upload the purple curry paste, mashing and stirring to soften it in the oil, about 1 minute.

2. Add the fowl and cook 1 to 2 minutes, tossing now and then to brown it lightly and mix it with the curry paste.

3. Add the coconut milk, bird broth, turmeric, soy sauce, sugar and salt and stir properly. Bring to a gentle boil and adjust heat to keep a lively simmer.

Four. Cook approximately 10 minutes till meat is cooked thru.

Five. Stir in lime juice, put off from warmth and cowl to hold curry heat at the same time as you put together the noodles.

6. Cook the noodles in a huge pot of hastily boiling water till smooth but nonetheless company, as little as 2 minutes for fresh noodles.

7. Drain, rinse properly in bloodless water, drain once more and divide the noodles among person serving bowls.

8. Ladle on hot curry, and sprinkle every serving with the shallots, cilantro, and green onions.

9. Serve hot and garnish in your taste.

16. Vegan Sweet Potato Falafels

The conventional center japanese dish falafel has been given a healthy makeover!

With the addition of turmeric and candy potato and by means of baking them inside the oven, this scrumptious gluten-unfastened, nutrition-stuffed vegan deal with can be enjoyed on a normal basis.

Ingredients:

- 1 can chickpeas

- 300g sweet potatoes

- 2 huge cloves garlic

- 1 handful fresh coriander leaves

- ¼ teaspoon floor cardamon

- 1 tablespoon of freshly grated turmeric

- 2 teaspoons ground coriander

- 1 teaspoon heaped floor cumin

- 2 tablespoons olive oil

- 1 teaspoon sea salt

- 2 tablespoons (+ a chunk greater for rolling with) chickpea flour

Instructions:

1.   Scrub and chop the sweet potato and boil till gentle with pores and skin nevertheless blanketed.

2.   Drain the candy potato and vicinity in a mixing bowl.

Three. Crush garlic and chop along with coriander leaves (as small as you may) with a pointy knife.

Four.   Add all elements into blender or food processor (besides for the gram flour).

5.   Blend till maximum of the mixture is broken down.

6.   Add the gram flour and retain to combine in with a spoon.

7.   Take a teaspoon of aggregate and roll into a golf ball sized ball.

Eight. Place on a gently oiled baking tray and bake in preheated oven at 400F for approximately 30 minutes or until tanned.

17. Turmeric-Garlic Shrimp With Cabbage and Mango Slaw

Ready in less than 30 minutes, this rapid shrimp dish is a unique manner to get your each day serving of turmeric.

Here's the way to make 4 servings:

Ingredients:

- 1 tbsp plus 1 tsp olive oil

- 2 limes, divided

- 1 tsp kosher salt

- 1/eight floor black pepper

- half of head purple cabbage, shredded (12 ouncestotal)

- 1 (8 oz.) mango, julienned

- 1/four small crimson onion, sliced into thin strips

- 2 tbsp clean chopped cilantro, divided

- 28 (1 lb peeled and deveined) greater large shrimp

- 2 garlic cloves, overwhelmed

- three/four tsp turmeric

- 1/four tsp cumin

- 1/8 tsp beaten pink pepper flakes

Instructions:

1. Combine 1 tbsp olive oil, juice of 1 lime, 3/4 tsp of the salt and pepper. Toss with the cabbage, purple onion, mango and 1 tbsp sparkling cilantro.

2. Combine shrimp with the last salt, turmeric, beaten purple pepper flakes, and cumin.

3. In a massive deep saute pan over medium-excessive warmness, upload 1/2 teaspoon of olive oil, and cook half of the shrimp 1 half to two minutes on each side, till shrimp is cooked thru and opaque.

4. Set aside, add the final half teaspoon of oil and ultimate shrimp and prepare dinner until shrimp is cooked through and opaque including the beaten garlic the remaining minute.

5. Return all the shrimp to the skillet, stir to mix with garlic.

6. Remove from warmth, squeeze lime over shrimp and toss with cilantro.

18. Cleansing Vegetable Turmeric Soup

If you're thinking about a detox, but don't recognise the way to detox deliciously, then let this vegetable turmeric soup help you. It will cleanse you from the inside out!

To make 4 servings:

Ingredients:

- 1 tablespoon olive oil

- 1 onion, diced

- 2 stalks celery, finely chopped

- 1 medium carrot, finely chopped

- 1 tablespoon floor turmeric

- 2 teaspoons garlic, minced (approximately four cloves)

- ½ teaspoon ground ginger

- ¼ teaspoon floor cayenne pepper

- 32 ounces vegetable broth

- 3-4 cups water

- 1 teaspoon salt, plus more to flavor

- ½ teaspoon black pepper, plus extra to flavor

- three cups cauliflower florets, chopped

- 1 15-ounce can blended beans, tired and rinsed

- 1 bunch kale, chopped

- One 7-ounce package shirataki noodles, drained

Instructions:

1. In a massive saucepan or pot over medium-low, heat oil.

2. Add onion and stir and prepare dinner for five-7 minutes, till the onions begin to brown.

3. Then, comprise carrots and celery and cook for three-5 greater mins, until the vegetables melt.

4. Add turmeric, garlic, ginger, and cayenne; stir till the veggies are coated.

5. Cook for 1 minute, till aromatic.

6. Add broth, water, salt, and pepper; stir. Bring to a boil; reduce warmth to low.

7. Add cauliflower, cowl and simmer for 10-15 mins, till cauliflower is tender.

8. When the cauliflower is fork gentle, add beans, kale, and noodles.

9. Cook until the kale is slightly wilted. Serve warm.

19. Watermelon Orange Ginger Turmeric Juice

If you're a turmeric lover, you'll adore this fruity, clean juice that's deliciously spiced up with the superfood.

For 4 servings:

Instructions:

- 18 oz.Freshly squeezed orange juice (from about 6 oranges)

- 7 cups of cubed watermelon

- Approx. Three" knob of peeled ginger root

- 3/four – 1 tsp ground turmeric

Instructions:

1. Juice six or so oranges, or until you've reached 18 ozof juice.

2. Cut and dice watermelon and add watermelon chunks to a blender.

3. Add ginger (no want to mince or grate) and turmeric.

4. Pour in orange juice.

5. Blend till watermelon chunks have liquefied and the juice is clean.

6. Pour juice through a strainer and discard pulp and ginger remnants.

7.   Serve.

20. Roasted Turmeric Cauliflower

You get flavor, convenience, and nutrition from this superfood powerhouse of a dish!

For 4 servings:

Ingredients :

- 1 head cauliflower

- 2 tablespoons coconut oil (melted)

- 1 teaspoon turmeric

- 1/2 teaspoon cumin

- half teaspoon beaten pink pepper

- 2 tablespoons water

- 1/2 teaspoon crushed garlic

- 2 tablespoons fresh basil (chopped)

Instructions:

1. Preheat oven to four hundred°F.

2. Chop the head of cauliflower into florets.

3.   Whisk together coconut oil, turmeric, cumin, crushed crimson pepper, garlic, and water.

4.   Place the cauliflower florets on a pan, pour the combination over them, and toss properly.

5.   Roast the cauliflower for half-hour, and pinnacle with clean basil.

21.Tropical Turmeric, Carrot, and Ginger Smoothie

This fast, easy, savory smoothie is packed full with goodness and delicious, adventurous flavors.

Not best will you experience the benefits of the fresh turmeric, however you'll be taking in at the least three of your five quantities of fruit and greens a day.

Here's the recipe for two servings:

Ingredients:

- 1 blood or navel orange, peel and pith removed

- 1 huge carrot, scrubbed and chopped

- ½ cup frozen mango chunks

- ⅔ cup coconut water

- 1 tablespoon shelled raw hemp seeds

- ¾ teaspoon finely grated peeled ginger

- 1½ teaspoons finely grated peeled turmeric

- Pinch of cayenne pepper

- Pinch of kosher salt

Instructions:

1.	Place all of your element in a blender.

2.	Purée until easy and stress if preferred.

3.   Drink without delay.

22. Turmeric & Coconut Roasted Butternut Squash Bisque

If you're seeking out to prepare soup that's also vegan and full of antioxidants and anti-inflammatories, this one pot wonder is the precise desire!

To make:

Ingredients:

- three medium size butternut squash

- 1 tablespoon of olive oil

- salt and pepper to taste

- three (15-ounce) cans of coconut milk

- 16 ounces of vegetable stock

- 1 tablespoon of chopped onion

- ½ teaspoon of cayenne pepper

- ½ teaspoon of ginger

- four teaspoons of turmeric

- ½ teaspoon garlic powder

- ½ teaspoon of salt

- 2 teaspoons of cinnamon

- ¼ teaspoon of cumin

- ¼ teaspoon of cloves

Instructions:

1.   Preheat the oven to four hundred levels Fahrenheit.

2.   Using a big knife, carefully cut the butternut squash in half lengthwise. Scoop out the seeds.

3.   Lay the butternut squash halves face up on a foil-coated baking sheet.

4.   Drizzle with olive oil, salt, and pepper.

5.   Roast in the oven for 1 hour, or until the squash is golden brown on the rims.

6.   Remove the squash from the oven and permit it rest until it's miles cool enough to address.

7.   Brown the onions in oil a big soup pot.

8.   Gently scoop the roasted butternut squash out of the pores and skin and into the pot. Discard the skin.

9.   Add the coconut milk and flip the heat to medium, permit the coconut milk and butternut squash to heat for 10 mins, stirring from time to time.

10.   Add the vegetable stock and all of the spices.

11.   Using an immersion blender, blend all the ingredients together until the soup is easy and creamy.

12.   Allow to cook dinner over medium heat for every other 30 minutes, stirring every so often.

13.   Serve warm, with clean bread.

23. Spiced Pancakes

These oil unfastened, first-rate fluffy vegan pancakes are a remarkable way of having your every day portion of turmeric into your day first aspect inside the morning.

To make 5-7 pancakes:

Ingredients:

- half cup unsweetened applesauce

- 1 1/four cup oat flour

- half of cup non-dairy milk

- 2 tbsps maple syrup

- 1 tbsp baking powder

- 1 tsp vanilla extract

- ½ tsp cinnamon

- ½ tsp ground turmeric

- pinch of black pepper

- ¼ tsp ginger

Instructions:

1.   Combine all components in a blender.

2.   Blend till blended. Don't over combination.

3.   Heat a non-stick skillet over medium-excessive warmth.

4.   Pour approximately 1/4 cup of batter into the pan. Since it's miles quite thick, spread/easy into a circle.

5.   Cook for two-three minutes on the primary facet. When you could without difficulty slide a spatula beneath, turn.

6.   Cook for every other 2-three minutes. Remove from pan.

7.   Repeat till all of the batter is long gone.

8.   To serve, top with yogurt, apple butter, and chopped nuts.

24. Golden Ginger & Turmeric Cookies

Vegan and gluten unfastened and definitely suitable for your cookies? Is it honestly possible? Absolutely!

Ingredients:

- half cup floor almonds

- 1 cups natural gluten loose oats

- half cup blended seeds

- 1 cup desiccated coconut

- Pinch red salt

- 1 tsp combined spice

- 1 tsp cinnamon

- three tsp ground ginger

- 1 knob sparkling ginger, grated

- 1 tsp sparkling turmeric grated or eleven/2 tsp ground turmeric

- 1/three cup maple syrup

- 1 tsp baking powder

- 1 ripe bananas, mashed

- half of cup melted coconut oil

- 2 tbsp almond butter

Instructions:

1.   Pre-warmness your oven to 400F.

2.   Mix all the dry elements in a massive bowl

3.   Melt the coconut oil in a saucepan (low heat) and then pour into a separate bowl, add within the bananas, maple syrup, almond butter, sparkling ginger, and turmeric – mix to mix everything.

4.   Add the wet components to the dry and mix simply nicely to mix the whole lot.

5.   Shape the mix into balls and dad them onto a covered baking tray.

6.   Bake for 20-25 minutes till slightly brown on the outdoor.

25. Turmeric Cake

This simple and delicious vegan turmeric cake is perfect to serve after dinner as a healthful dessert opportunity.

Here's the way to make it:

Ingredients:

- three cups self-rising flour

- ⅔ cup sugar

- 1 tbsp turmeric

- 1 ½ cups unsweetened shredded coconut

- Pinch of salt

- ¾ cup coconut oil

- 1 ¾ cups coconut milk

- 1 tbsp tahini (sesame paste)

- Shelled pistachios for garnish

Instructions:

1. Preheat the oven to 350F

2. Coat the lowest and sides of an eleven×7 in baking dish with tahini

3. In a massive bowl, integrate flour, sugar, turmeric and shredded coconut and salt. Mix nicely.

4.   Add coconut oil and milk and lightly stir all of the elements together till just mixed (do not overmix).

5.   Spoon batter lightly at the organized baking dish.

6.   Decorate with pistachios on pinnacle and bake at 350F for about 45 minutes.

7.   Let sit for as a minimum 15 mins earlier than slicing.

26. Turmeric Chickpea Fritters

Mouth-wateringly gentle at the interior however with a great crunch on the outdoor, those hearty, garlicky, clean chickpea fritters are infused with the marvel spice.

Ingredients:

Chickpea Fritters:

- 1 flax egg (1 tbsp flaxseed meal + 2.Five tbsp water)

- 1-2 tbsp olive oil, divided (plus extra for sautéing)

- 4 cloves garlic, minced

- half cup panko bread crumbs

- 1/4 cup sparkling parsley, finely chopped

- three tbsp parmesan cheese

- 1 tbsp hulled white sesame seeds or hemp seeds

- 2 tsp coconut sugar

- half tsp floor turmeric

- 1 half of tsp floor cumin

- Pinch sea salt and black pepper

- 1/2 lemon, juiced

- 1 15-ounce can chickpeas, tired, rinsed and carefully dried

For The Coating:

- 2 tbsp parmesan cheese

- 3 Tbsp (12 g) panko bread crumbs

To Prepare

1.   Preheat oven to 375 tiers and add flax egg to a food processor or high-velocity blender.

2.   Heat a large metallic or cast iron skillet over medium warmness.

3.   Once hot, add 1 Tbsp (15 ml) olive oil and minced garlic. Sauté until slightly browned, stirring frequently – about three minutes.

4.   Remove from warmth and funky barely, then add to food processor or blender with a flax egg.

5.   Add panko bread crumbs, parsley, parmesan cheese, sesame seeds (elective), coconut sugar, turmeric, cumin, a pinch every salt + pepper, and 1 tsp olive oil, and lemon juice.

6.   Pulse/mixture till small bits continue to be, scraping down sides as needed.

7.   Add rinsed/dried chickpeas and blend till a "dough" is fashioned, scraping down acets as needed. You don't need the chickpeas to turn into a paste, however you furthermore may don't want any left whole.

8.   Taste and adjust seasonings as needed.

9.   To make the coating, mix parmesan cheese and panko breadcrumbs in a shallow bowl. Set aside.

10.   Scoop out heaping 1 Tbsp quantities of dough, shape/roll into balls – about 15 general.

1.   Roll fritters in the vegan parmesan cheese-panko bread crumb aggregate to coat.

2.   Heat the identical skillet you used in advance over medium warmness.

13.   Once warm, upload sufficient oil to form a thin layer on the lowest of the skillet, then upload fritters. Depending on the size of your pan, you may need to prepare dinner them in two batches as to now not crowd the pan. Add extra oil as needed.

14.   Brown fritters for 4-5 minutes total, shaking the pan to roll them around and brown all sides. Turn down the warmth slightly if browning too fast.

15.   Add sautéed fritters to a bare or foil-coated baking sheet and transfer to the preheated oven and bake for 12-15 mins.

16.   Once fritters are golden brown and fairly firm to the touch, do away with from oven. Let cool a couple of minutes before serving. They will firm up the longer they cool.

27. Raw Vegan Ginger And Turmeric Cheesecakes

If you've got a sweet tooth and would just like to devour cake each day without feeling guilty for doing so, these turmeric cheesecakes could be exactly the one you're looking for.

Ingredients:

For the bottom:

- 100g almonds

- 90g dates

For the filling:

- 250g cashews

- 20g softened coconut butter

- 50g melted coconut oil

- 10g fresh ginger

- 10g sparkling turmeric

- 30g lemon juice

- 75g maple syrup

- 1 cup water

For the caramel:

- 50g dates

- 15g melted coconut oil

- 8g sparkling ginger

- half cup water

Instructions:

1.   Add the ingredients for the base to a blender and blitz till you get a sticky, crumbly blend.

2.   Press the combination into your mini cheesecake molds. You can also make one large cake.

3.   Add the ginger, turmeric, lemon juice and water to a blender and blitz until you absolutely mix the whole thing – you must now not have any peculiar bits and pieces or chunks of ginger or turmeric left.

4.   Add the rest of the ingredients for the filling and procedure till you get a outstanding easy, silky cream.

5.   Spoon this onto the bases and dad it into the refrigerator (or freezer) to set.

6.   To make the caramel, upload the components to a blender and technique for an excellent minute or till you get it as clean as possible. That must be exceedingly mild and smooth.

7.   Spoon the caramel on top of the cheesecakes whilst prepared to serve.

 By adopting a number of these easy turmeric recipes into your life, you may begin to live a fuller, healthier and tastier life.

Disclaimer

The information contained on this book is intended for educational purposes only and is not a substitute for advice, diagnosis or treatment by a licensed physician.

It is not meant to cover all possible precautions, drug interactions, circumstances or adverse effects.

You should seek prompt medical care for any health issues and consult your doctor before using alternative medicine or making a change to your regime

About The Author

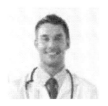

Biography

Dr. M. kotb is a board certified internist

Dr. Kotb is also medical director of the ELITE medical Center for internal medicine and Nutrition Studies,

which promotes

optimal nutrition through science-based education, advocacy,

and research in partnership with Hanover University, Germany

As medical director and chief medical editor at the training program of physicians, He now oversees a team of staff physicians and medical reviewers UK.

Responsible for creating content and assuring its continued medical accuracy and relevance

Dr. Kotb is a regular expert on national and local broadcast media, including regular appearances on UK Channels

He has also been interviewed by local and nationally syndicated radio stations, magazines, and newspapers across the country, speaking on everything from hangover remedies to navigating the Internet for accurate, credible health information.

Dr. Kotb serves as a member of the Nutrition Wellness Educator Certification Panel, established by the U.K. Association of Family Services.

The panel is responsible for determining the competency scope of the Nutrition Educator certification.

Dr. Kotb also volunteers at the Good medicine Health Center in Berkshire, where he sees patients who do not have health insurance or are unable to pay for health care.

As a board-certified internist, Dr. Kotb's interest and knowledge span a wide array of medical topics.

He is particularly interested in prevention and helping people live a healthy, active lifestyle

Dr. Kotb is a member of the international association of liver disease

He is A pioneer and internationally recognized expert in the fields of INTERVENTIONAL HEPATOLOGY,

DR M KOTB, MD is the creator of Be EXCELLENT, a proprietary brand of health coaching BOOKS.

He is A U.K. bestselling author WITH MORE than 200 books

He had been invited for over 150 oral presentations in conferences focusing primarily on family medicine

He is the Vice president of Berkshire charity for orphans.

Learn more about DR KOTB at

https://www.amazon.com/Dr-Kotb/e/B078H598L5

You can discover his facebook fan page here ==>

https://www.facebook.com/Neverseenbefore.co.uk/

you can join his email list here ==>

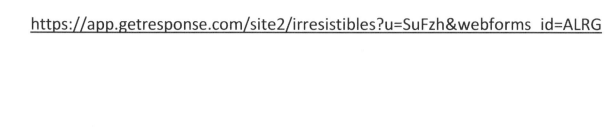

https://app.getresponse.com/site2/irresistibles?u=SuFzh&webforms_id=ALRG

For correspondence :

London

Address Line1: House Old Bath Road Colnbrook

Address Line2: JED 769904

City: Slough

State: Berkshire

ZipCode: SL3 0NS

Tel: 01753-210399

Other Books By DR KOTB

HOW TO BEAT THE KRYPTONITE: The proven 12 steps protocol from the top successful ADHD superwomen to sister, wife, mother with ADHD to harmonize brain

http://amzn.to/2BxzGWf

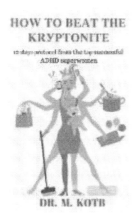

Brain Rules For Panic Sons : A 99 Proven Ways To Relief Panic Attacks, Harmonize Your Brain Anxiety And Rebuild Your Relationships At Home And Work

http://amzn.to/2D2fT0L

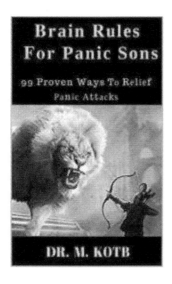

The Regretful butterfly: 100 Worst Mistakes you may make in your hypothyroidism solution protocol

http://amzn.to/2BUfYEo

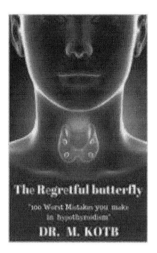

THE FIBROMYALGIA-REVERSAL PROGRAM (MADE EASY) :The New Scientifically Proven Therapy To fix Fibromyalgia pain And reverse Chronic Fatigue In 6 Weeks

http://amzn.to/2BWblo1

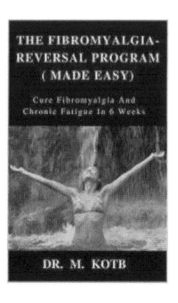

One Last Thing...

If you enjoyed this book or found it useful I'd be very grateful if you'd post a short review on Amazon.

Your support really does make a difference and I read all the reviews personally so I can get your feedback and make this book even better.

Thanks again for your support!

Made in the USA
Lexington, KY
17 June 2018